Calories Count
The Truth About Losing Weight

By

Jessica Cleary

1663 LIBERTY DRIVE, SUITE 200
BLOOMINGTON, INDIANA 47403
(800) 839-8640
WWW.AUTHORHOUSE.COM

First published by AuthorHouse 12/29/04

ISBN: 1-4184-9176-4 (e)
ISBN: 1-4184-9175-6 (sc)

Printed in the United States of America
Bloomington, Indiana

This book is printed on acid-free paper.

Table of Contents

Introduction

I would like to introduce this book with a story from an author by the name of Brillat-Savarin. He wrote a book titled *The Physiology of Taste* in 1825. Brillat-Savarin wrote on the subject of gastronomy, which is the study or art of good eating. He was a brilliant man, a lawyer by profession, and a member of the Court of Appeals in Paris. In 1825 he published at his own expense *The Physiology of Taste*, a book on which he had been working with amusement and pleasure for some decades. This is quite apropos given that I have been working on this book for many years as well, also with amusement and pleasure. It does not take a scientist to enjoy the pleasures of good eating, but it takes understanding the purpose food plays in your life and how to enjoy it in moderation, as anything can be enjoyed in minimum amounts.

I shall begin with a story, which proves that it takes real courage to lose weight or to keep from gaining.

M. Louis Greffulhe, who was later honored by His Majesty with the title of Count, came to see me one morning and told me he understood that I was interested in the subject of obesity, and that since he was in grave danger of it, he wished my advice.

"Sir," I said to him, "since I am not a graduate doctor, I would be within my right to refuse to counsel you. However, I am at your command, but on a single condition: that you will give me your word of honor to follow, for one month, and with the greatest fidelity, the rules of conduct that I shall prescribe for you."

M. Greffulhe made the promise I demanded. We shook hands on it, and the very next day I asked him to weigh himself at the beginning and at the end of the treatment so that we might have a mathematical basis on which to judge the results.

One month later, M. Greffulhe returned to see me and spoke to me in much the following terms:

"Sir, I have followed your prescription as faithfully as if my life depended on it, and I have verified the fact that my weight has gone down by some three pounds, or even a little more. But, in order to achieve this, I have suffered so much that, while I offer you all my thanks for your excellent advice, I must renounce what good it might do for me and abandon myself in the future to whatever providence has in store."

After this decision, which I did not hear without real distress, the inevitable occurred. M. Greffulhe became even more obese, was the victim of all inconveniences of extreme corpulence, and, when he was barely forty years old, died as the result of an asthmatic condition to which he became subject.

The main purpose of this book is to serve as a guide or reference to attaining your lifelong nutritional needs. The book contains facts about food that should not change with time. I will teach you to calculate your own caloric intake via a famous equation as well as teach you where to get the essential nutrients your body needs and how to maintain an ideal body weight throughout your lifetime.

I divide this book into several key chapters, all short but significant. I'll first explain the calculation and then where your nutrient sources are found. The following chapters are then broken up into the major nutrient groups beginning with water. In the last several chapters, I discuss diabetes, cholesterol/fat, and alcohol.

I will quote for you again from the book *The Physiology of Taste* some words I think are quite eloquently stated on the nature of taste.

Because taste as Nature has endowed us with is still one of our senses which gives us the greatest joy......

Because the pleasure of eating is only
one which, indulged in moderately; is not
followed by regret;

Because it is common to all periods in history, all
ages of man, and all social conditions;

Because it recurs of necessity at least once
every day, and can be repeated without
inconvenience two to three times in the
space of hours;

Because it can mingle with all other pleasures,
and
even console us for their absence;

Because its sensations are at once more lasting
than
others and more subject to our will;

Because, finally, in eating we experience a certain
special and indefinable well-being, which arises

from our instinctive realization that by the very act we perform we are repairing our bodily losses and prolonging our lives.

Hunger-

1: a strong desire for food 2: a: the weakness, debilitation, or pain caused by prolonged lack of food, starvation b: mild discomfort or uneasy sensation caused by lack of food 3: a strong desire or craving for anything; a hunger for affection

Taste-

1: to distinguish the flavor of by taking into the mouth 2: to eat or drink a small quantity of 3: to distinguish flavors in the mouth; to have an experience; to have a distinct flavor

Appetite-

1: any of the instinctive desires to keep up organic life; especially, the desire to eat 2: a: an inherent craving b: taste, preference

5 Rules to Remember

1. Eat from the five food groups (i.e., protein, fruits, vegetables, fat, and carbohydrates).

2. Limit your carbohydrate intake.

3. Exercise.

4. Watch your total calories every day.

5. Drink water, and watch out for unnecessary calories from Drinking alcohol. Drinking lots of alcohol adds lots of unwanted calories to your day.

Reminder: Eating just 100 calories more than you need each day can lead to a 10-pound weight gain in a year. That is how easy it is.

Chapter 1:
Designing Your Diet

Calculate Your Caloric Intake

Based upon the idea that everyone has his or her
own metabolic makeup, and with the new field of
nutrigenomics, everyone must learn to eat for him- or
herself. We are all different shapes and sizes. Now
you can calculate on your own just how much you
should be eating (calorically) based upon your weight,
height, and activity level.

This calculation is used currently in hospitals by
dietitians and doctors to determine (via estimation
based upon an individual's metabolic rate) just how

many calories one should be receiving either via tube or by mouth. I believe this idea can be extrapolated to teach you, and those who wish to stay healthy for a lifetime, to calculate your caloric needs based upon your own body makeup. No one knows your body better than you. By knowing just how much to eat daily and learning what your foods are composed of, you can prevent the ever-present 10-pound-weight-gain-in-a-year phenomenon. By eating just 100 calories more each day over the span of a year, you can put on 10 pounds easily, especially if you are not exercising.

You can use this estimation of caloric intake throughout your lifetime. By maintaining a healthy weight throughout your life, you can prevent some very devastating diseases from occurring. Whether you are a child or an adult, it is never too late to focus on your intake and activity levels. Today, children are getting diseases we used to only see adults get. The foods you eat can affect your mind and body. There are few times in your life when your caloric needs may vary. These times include when you are young and growing, if you are a pregnant woman, if you are lactating, or if you are a sick person healing from wounds. Other than these times, knowing what and how much to ingest can save you from lifelong illnesses.

Estimation of Caloric Intake

Your basal metabolism is your metabolism at rest. Everyone has a different metabolism depending on lifestyle. For example, a professional runner has a higher metabolism than a computer programmer, who may exercise little, if at all. This difference in metabolism may directly affect how you lose or gain weight.

By using the following equation, we can determine just how many calories one requires to either maintain, gain, or lose weight. Using one's basal metabolic rate, we can make this calculation using a close estimation of just how much one needs to eat based on one's individual metabolism. Your friend's metabolism might be different from yours.

The following equation is used in the clinical setting to determine caloric intake for patients such as those requiring tube feeding as well as those in the general population. Calories are important to know about.

The following equation can be used to determine weight loss or gain as well as a maintenance caloric intake amount. Everyone should have an idea of just how much they should be eating daily to maintain a healthy weight for a lifetime.

How to use this book:

You will learn how to calculate your caloric intake based upon your desirable weight range. For example, if you are a 165–pound, 5' 5" female, your ideal weight should be around 125 pounds. You would then use your ideal weight as your desirable weight in the calculation.

The ideal weight guide is provided to give you an idea of a healthy weight range for you to maintain throughout your adult life. Everyone has a different body structure, so this is just to give you an estimation of the range where you ought to be. Watching your total calories daily can help you reach your weight-loss goals. This requires discipline and patience, but it pays off.

How to Calculate Your Energy Needs

Basal Energy Expenditure (BEE)
To calculate energy expenditure or calories necessary per day, the Harris Benedict equations are used and are based on 167 men and 103 women aged 15 to 74 with a body mass index (BMI) range of 12.3 to 32.5. Indirect calorimetry was used to estimate energy expenditure, not always under truly basal conditions. These BEE equations generally overestimate BEE by 15 percent to 15 percent.

The totals equal the total kilocalories per day one should eat to reach a goal or maintain an ideal weight.

Everyone is different. For example, some people exercise more and burn more calories and therefore require more calories to maintain their weight. The main idea is that calories taken in should equal calories burned for maintaining optimal weight. For losing weight, the equation should be calories taken in are less than calories burned, and this includes your body's energy requirements just to exist.

Estimating Your Ideal Body Weight

Energy balance is the essence of eating well. If
you eat too much, you gain weight. If you eat just
right, you maintain. And if you eat less than what is
necessary to maintain, you lose weight. Many people
gain weight over time by eating just a little more than
necessary each day, which can lead to a weight gain
over time. This equates to how many kilocalories
(calories) one should eat per day. A kilocalorie, also
usually recognized as calories, is a unit of measure for
energy produced in the body by the energy yielding
macronutrients, carbohydrates, fats, and protein. All
three macronutrients in our food can be metabolized
to yield body energy.

Use the following equation to calculate your energy
balance, which is an estimate of basal energy
expenditure (BEE). It is calculated from special data.

For Men:

$$BEE = 66 + (13.7 \times W) + (5 \times H) - (6.8 \times A) =$$

For Women:

$$BEE = 665 + (9.6 \times W) + (1.8 \times H) - (4.7 \times A) =$$

W = kg body weight

H = height in cm

A = age in years

The following are helpful conversions:

There are 2.54cm/inch for the height conversion.

There are 2.2kg/lb for the weight conversion.

For example, a 135-lb. woman weighs 61 kg.

135 lb. divided by 2.2kg/lb = 61 kg

An example for the conversion of feet to centimeters:

A 5' 7" person is 67 inches tall.

Multiply 67 in. x 2.54cm/in. = 170cm

Ideal Body Weight Chart

WOMEN'S HEIGHT			MEN'S HEIGHT		
4'10"	—	90 lb	4'10"	—	94 lb
4'11"	—	95 lb	4'11"	—	100 lb
5'0"	—	100 lb	5'0"	—	106 lb
5'1"	—	105 lb	5'1"	—	112 lb
5'2"	—	110 lb	5'2"	—	118 lb
5'3"	—	115 lb	5'3"	—	124 lb
5'4"	—	120 lb	5'4"	—	130 lb
5'5"	—	125 lb	5'5"	—	136 lb
5'6"	—	130 lb	5'6"	—	142 lb
5'7"	—	135 lb	5'7"	—	148 lb
5'8"	—	140 lb	5'8"	—	154 lb
5'9"	—	145 lb	5'9"	—	160 lb
5'10"	—	150 lb	5'10"	—	166 lb
5'11"	—	155 lb	5'11"	—	172 lb
6'0"	—	160 lb	6'0"	—	178 lb
6'1"	—	165 lb	6'1"	—	184 lb
6'2"	—	170 lb	6'2"	—	190 lb
ADD 5 LB FOR EVERY INCH			ADD 6 LB FOR EVERY INCH		

Chapter 2: Water

Water-

Water is found wherever there are animals. It sometimes takes the place of milk for adults, and it is as necessary to us as the air we breathe.

Seventy percent of the body is made up of water. Our muscles hold most of it. Water's role in our existence is so expansive and significant that our lives depend on the abundance of this incredible compound. Significant reactions take place in water in our blood, our cells, and our intracellular as well as extracellular space. All cells require water to maintain adequate structure. Without water there would be little growth. Try to drink at least 32 oz. to 64 oz. per day unless otherwise stated.

Are you wondering what the benefits of drinking so much water are? The following lists what water does for you.

1. Water can suppress your appetite naturally and help metabolize stored fat.

2. Drinking enough water is the best treatment for fluid retention unless medically recommended otherwise. Watch your salt intake–talk about fluid retention!

3. Water helps maintain proper muscle tone.

4. Water helps rid the body of waste. Basically, water can relieve constipation if you drink it on a regular basis. Shoot for drinking the same amount daily.

Chapter 3: Protein

Protein-

Protein is one of the three sources of energy from food. Proteins are the basic substance of the body and are found in every cell. Half of your body is made up of protein; the other half is water. Protein is essential for healthy muscle, bone, cartilage, blood, and your skin as well as your immune system (the lymphatic system). Protein is made up of amino acids, which form hundreds of different proteins used by the body.

How much protein do you really need? There is a general rule or guideline to go by for protein needs. For example, if you are trying to put on weight or build muscle, you would need to eat more protein as well as do weight training. If you are trying to meet your daily needs, the following guideline can be followed:

Children (7-10 years old)	37 gms of protein
Adolescent females	46 gms of protein
Adolescent males (remember	56 gms of protein
	children are growing)
Adults	44 gms of protein
Pregnancy	add 30 gms of protein
Nursing	add 20 gms of protein

Protein is essential for healthy muscle, bone, cartilage, lymphatic system, blood, and skin. Protein is made up of building blocks called amino acids, which link together in different sequences to form hundreds of different proteins used by the body.

When excess protein is broken down in the body, part is stored as fat; another part is converted to nitrogen and is flushed out by the kidneys.

There is speculation that too much meat protein, such as red meat, as well as dietary fat, may be implicated in clogged arteries, heart disease, and high blood pressure. Most experts still believe, however, that the fat in foods is the main enemy of the cardiovascular system. I believe this, in conjunction with the amount of calories consumed, can contribute to serious heart problems.

The following are examples of complete proteins:
cereal with milk
legumes with rice, wheat, corn or barley
spaghetti with sauce containing a little lean ground beef or grated cheese

In this chapter, I will discuss where to find protein, and I will give you an estimate of its caloric value as well as the amount of protein present in each source. These are all important pieces of information in attaining optimal nutrition. I will break this chapter up into four groups: animal protein (such as meat and chicken); fish and seafood; dairy (including eggs);

and legumes and nuts. These four groups represent great sources of protein.

Animal Protein

Animal protein, such as a 3.5-oz. chicken breast, for example, contains around 23 grams of protein and about 125 calories. Generally this size portion of animal protein will contain around the same amount of protein and calories, but the meats will vary mostly in fat content.

The following is a list of sources of protein from animals as well as birds.
Chicken
Capon
Turkey
Beef
Lamb
Ham (a.k.a. pig)
Veal
Salami
Liverwurst
Duck
Ostrich
Goose
Quail

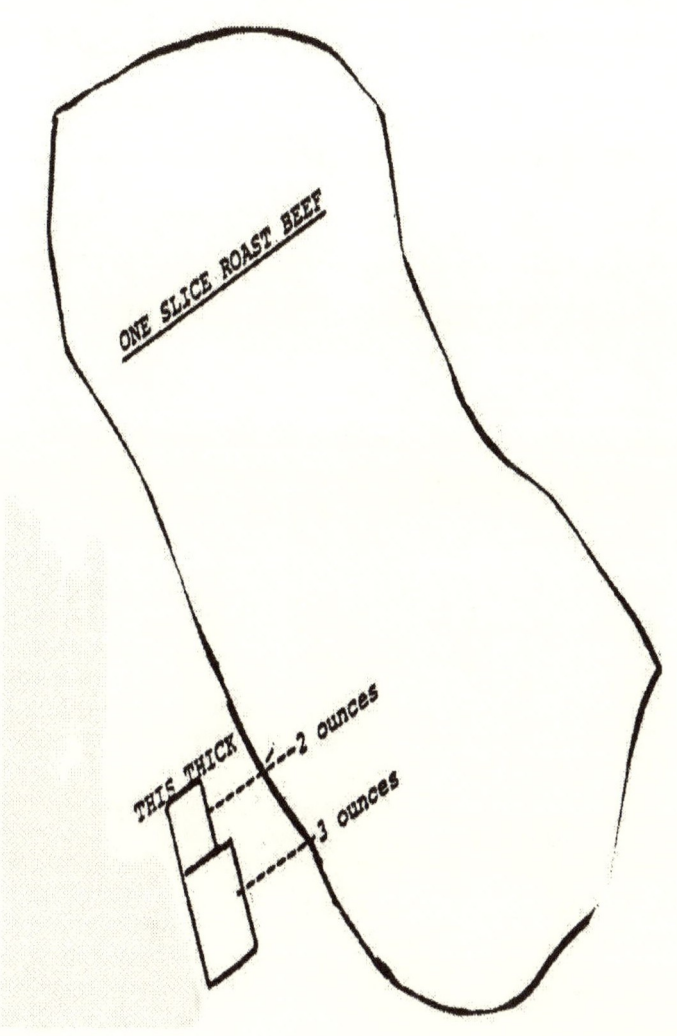

ONE SLICE ROAST BEEF

THIS THICK ---2 ounces

---3 ounces

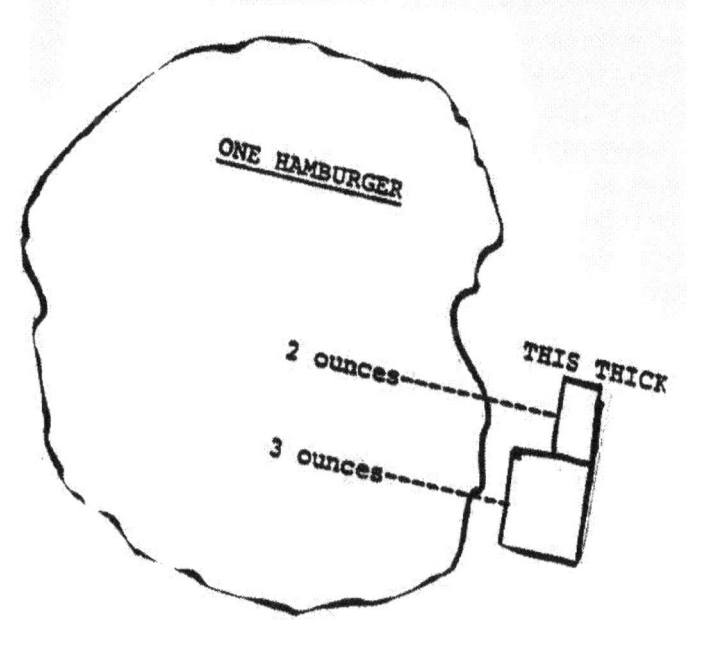

ONE HAMBURGER

2 ounces- - - - - - - THIS THICK

3 ounces- - - - - -

The following is a list of game as well as other animals sometimes eaten. They are listed in order of lean to fattiest.

Like chicken, a 3.5-oz. portion size may contain around 125 calories. An example of a 2- to 3-oz. portion is shown by the drawings.

Antelope	Caribou
Goat	Squirrel
Bison	Beefalo
Water Buffalo	Beaver
Turtle	Eel
Frog Legs	Horse
Moose	Opossum
Rabbit	Raccoon
Snail	Muskrat
Boar	Bear
Whale meat	

Fish and Seafood

Fish are a great source of protein. I have listed the following from lean to fatty, beginning with the leanest. I also include a drawing to show visually what a 2- to 3-oz. portion looks like for times when you need to eye your portion size (especially when eating out).

One 3-oz. serving of fish can range between 80 and 160 calories, depending on the kind of fish.

Lean

Cod (extremely lean)	Sea Bass
Pike	Whiting
Clams	Oysters
Squid	Haddock
Scallops	

Moderately Lean

Bluefin	Tuna
Halibut	Mullet
Red Snapper	Swordfish
Crab	Crayfish
Lobster	Shrimp

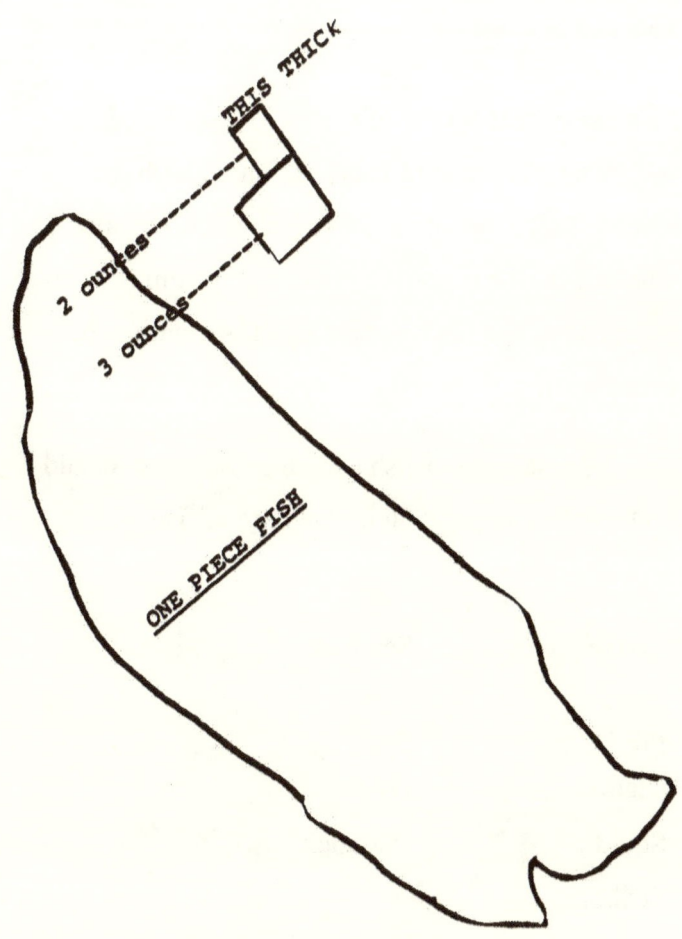

Fatty, but some of these are excellent sources of omega-3 fatty acids (linoleic acids)

Salmon	Albacore Tuna
Mackerel	Herring
Shad	Trout

Dairy

Dairy products are also an excellent source of protein as well as providing calcium. Some ways to achieve your protein needs can be met through dairy products such as those discussed below. Dairy products vary in fat content, but they often remain consistent with their protein content. The first example shows the caloric difference in milk but you can see that the protein remains almost the same. Fat content varies as well.

Vitamin D

whole milk (8 oz.)	151 calories	8 grams protein
2% low-fat milk	121 calories	9 grams protein
1% milk	100 calories	9 grams protein
Skim milk	90 calories	8-9 grams protein

| 2% low-fat cottage cheese (1/2 cup) | 90 calories | 14 grams protein |
| nonfat cottage cheese | 90 calories | 14 grams protein |

| nonfat yogurt (16 oz.) | 100 calories | 10 grams protein |

Regular yogurt (not nonfat) 270 calories   10 grams protein

| 1 egg | 70 calories | 8 grams protein |
| 1 egg white | 16 calories | 3 grams protein |

The idea is to get the most nutrients possible out of the food you eat.

The following list consists of different kinds of cheeses, which, on average, contain between 85 and 110 calories per 1-oz. serving.

American	Blue
Brick	Brie
Camembert	Caraway
Cheddar	Cheshire
Colby	Edam
Feta	Fontina
Gjetost	Goat (8-9 gms protein)
Gouda	Gruyere
Havarti	Jalapeno Jack
Mozzarella (part-skim, low-moisture is highest in protein)	
Muenster	Neufchatel
Parmesan	Pimento
Port du Salut	Provolone
Ricotta	Romano
Roquefo	rt (made from sheep's milk)
Swiss	Tilsit

Eggs

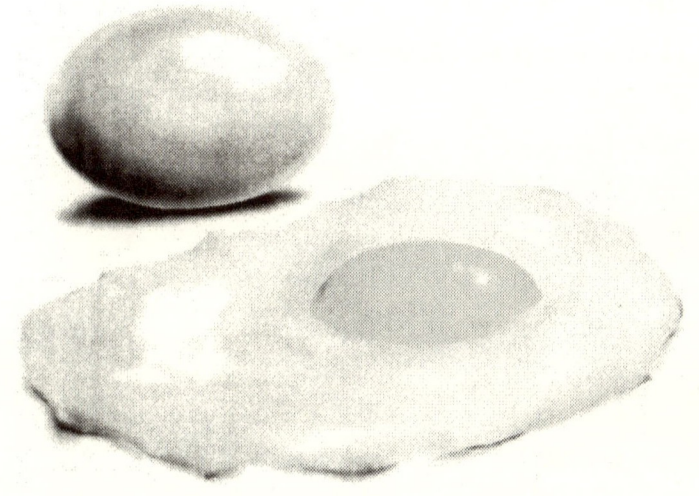

What is all the fuss about? People who love eggs may already know that they happen to contain the highest quality protein that exists. So why such a bad rap? In fact eggs are really not so bad for you after all. There exists much confusion concerning the humble egg, but aside from the fact that one egg alone contains 272 milligrams of cholesterol, I cannot think of one bad thing about them. The egg just happens to be infamous for the amount of cholesterol it naturally contains. A goose egg contains around 1,200 milligrams of cholesterol, but you do not hear anyone bad-rapping the poor goose egg.

If it is necessary for you to watch your cholesterol intake, then you should not be eating a dozen eggs a week. But you should also be monitoring your total caloric intake as well as your fat intake. Overeating affects your cholesterol levels as well. You can take Lipitor or other cholesterol-lowering medications, but in the end, it is up to you to watch your intake of any harmful substances. If you are genetically disposed to high cholesterol, there's often nothing you can do about it other than avoid all cholesterol-containing foods and hope your cholesterol levels go down. But even then there is no guarantee that it will. Cholesterol-lowering drugs do work wonders these days though. But you cannot just rely on these drugs alone. By just cutting out eggs rather than cutting down on high-fat foods, you are losing out on a very nutritious staple. In general, you want to watch your overall fat intake, not just foods high in cholesterol. Cholesterol buildup in your arteries blocks blood from passing through, thereby inhibiting oxygenated blood and essential nutrients from reaching their destination. As I stated before, we cannot blame this effect all on the poor egg because a high-fat diet contributes to this very dangerous buildup as well. I cannot say this enough times. The idea is to try to keep your arteries clean. Like drainage pipes when it rains, leaves from the year before have a tendency to block water from passing through, and it is this buildup of leaves like lipids that leads to blocked passageways. So please keep your arteries clean as much as possible. Bypass surgery is not to be considered like plastic surgery.

Back to eggs and why I highly recommend them. How they ever got to be considered "dangerous" or "bad" I'll never understand. So you may ask, what is so great about eggs then? Well, I will tell you. Yes, eggs contain the highest quality protein, 22 essential amino acids in all–it's a complete protein. All 22 are required for optimal nutrition, but eggs also contain a very important vitamin: vitamin A. Protein is important in helping us grow and repair our bodies; vitamin A promotes good vision and helps form and maintain healthy skin. Vitamin A is also known as one of the antioxidants (a fat-soluble vitamin) and may also help to protect against some cancers.

Sounds pretty good, so how did we lose sight of such a wonderful food? Eggs are such a lovely source of both protein and vitamin A. An excellent way to remember good sources of vitamin A is to think of the colors orange and green, which are found in carrots and spinach. Foods with these deep colors generally contain excellent sources of vitamin A as well as several other essential vitamins.

The yellow of the egg yolk contains all the cholesterol and fat, but it also contains vitamin A. One egg contains a total of 6.1 grams of high-quality protein and 93.8 RE of vitamin A. The recommended daily allowance (RDA) for vitamin A for an adult female is 800 RE; the RDA for males is 1,000 RE.

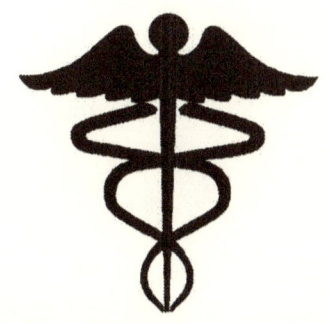

Egg Stats

79 calories

6.1 grams of protein

5.6 grams of fat

272 milligrams of cholesterol

The yolk, however, does contain the majority of the calories, totaling around 63. It also contains 2.8 grams of protein and 5.6 grams of fat. And last but not least, it contains those infamous 272 milligrams of cholesterol. The white holds its own by containing 16 calories and 3.3 grams of protein. So you can see that the white of the egg still holds its fair share of protein. But if you are told you must watch your cholesterol intake, you can still eat egg whites– just watch out for the yolk. Scramble up a few egg whites for breakfast– my grandpa does, and he is 88 years old and in phenomenal shape. I am incredibly proud of him. He scrambles up a few egg whites for breakfast most mornings.

My thought on the egg is to look at the sunny-side up side, and view it for its benefits. The egg provides an excellent source of protein and a completely natural source of vitamin A. To those vegetarians out there, please remember the little (or not so little) egg when you are shopping or cooking. Also note that the egg has been around for centuries. The Romans, French, Chinese, Japanese, Koreans as well as

Russians have used eggs in their diets and on their tables for many years, if not for centuries, as both a staple and a delicacy.

Let us not forget that eggs are in almost every baking recipe that exists as well as in many cooking recipes and salad dressings (Caesar salad, for example). A cookie would not be a cookie and angel food cake would not exist without eggs. It is not called angel food cake for nothing. Which came first, the chicken or the egg? Or does it really matter? So don't be a chicken when it comes to eating 'em.

Legumes

Beans are another good source of protein for non-meat eaters, although eggs are considered the highest quality protein because they contain all the essential amino acids that are required for optimal nutrition as well as for growth requirements. Complete protein is necessary for proper nutrition. Plant proteins are not considered complete. Animal proteins are complete, however. Therefore plant proteins need to be combined with grains to be considered complete.

1 serving of beans (8 oz.) ranges from 182 to 285 calories. Typically, beans have 11-12 grams of protein per serving. For example, 8 oz. of kidney beans contains 285 calories and about 12 grams of protein. Garbanzo beans, on the other hand, are similar but higher in fat. Generally, beans tend to be low in fat.

Lentil	Kidney
Pinto	Lima
Butter	Black
Garbanzo	Turtle
Fava (highest in protein at about 14 grams)	Mung
Navy	Hyacinth

Nuts

Nuts are also an excellent source of protein. Nuts are not only a good source of protein, they also contain nutrients such as folate, potassium, and magnesium. Although nuts contain a significant amount of fat, they are a good source of polyunsaturated fat without cholesterol. Nuts are cholesterol-free. Plants in general are cholesterol-free.

For example, 2 tablespoons of peanut butter have 190 calories, 7 grams of protein, and 16 grams of fat. Peanut butter may contain sugar if it is not all-natural because that is how they make it today. Nuts by themselves contain only protein and fat.

The following is a list of nuts that may be familiar to you. They are a good snack choice for those who are looking for extra protein.

One ounce of nuts, which is equivalent to about a handful, contains around 150 calories, between 13 and 15 grams of fat, and about 4 grams of protein.

Almonds	Pili nuts
Beechnuts	Pinenuts
Brazil nuts	Pistachios
Butternuts	Sesame seeds
Cashews	Sunflowers
Filberts	Walnuts
Ginko nuts	Watermelon (8 grams of protein per oz.)
Macadamias	Peanuts

Chapter 4: Fat

Fat-

Fat is a source of essential fatty acids, which help keep the body alive. Fats give the body structure, are a carrier of fat-soluble vitamins (A, D, E, and K), and are necessary for many metabolic functions.

Dietary fat is considered the number one nutritional danger.

Dietary fat is a term used to encompass a variety of different kinds of fats and oils found in foods. Fats are a concentrated source of energy, a source of essential fatty acids that help keep the body alive. For example, salmon is an excellent source of a good fat called omega-3 fatty acid (an unsaturated fat), which is also called eicosapentaenoic acid (EPA). Many scientists suspect that the active heart-protective agent in fish is EPA.

Types of Fat

There are two types of fat: unsaturated fat and saturated.

Saturated Fat-
is the type that leads to damaged arteries and is found in animal-derived foods such as meat and dairy products.

Unsaturated Fats-
are good for the arteries. These are the ones found in fish and most vegetable oils such as corn oil, soybean oil, safflower oil, and sunflower oils. These oils help lower blood cholesterol.

Where we get fat in the diet:

Meat	Dairy, eggs
Fats, oils	Desserts, snacks
Breads, grains, potatoes (as in french fries, of course)	
Nuts, beans	Miscellaneous Items

The most fat comes from hamburgers and meatloaf unless you use a very lean source of meat. Next in line are hot dogs, ham and luncheon meats, whole milk, doughnuts, cakes and cookies, and beef steaks and roasts.

Why Do We Need Fat?

1. Fat provides energy storage.

2. It provides energy to the body.

3. Fat gives us a feeling of satiety (a feeling of fullness).

4. It transports fat-soluble vitamins during absorption from the intestines.

6. Fat insulates and protects the body.

7. It forms eicosanoids from linoleic and linolenic fatty acids.

Fat Deficiency

How Much Fat Do We Actually Need to Eat to Prevent a Deficiency?
Is There Such a Thing?

To prevent a deficiency of fat, we need to take in the equivalent of one tablespoon of vegetable oil per day to obtain the essential fatty acids. Most of us eat at least this much daily via the foods we eat, either from fish, meat, or other foods. Very few Americans become fatty acid deficient.

Fat Consumption and Disease: What's the Connection?

Several studies have shown a correlation between coronary heart disease, blood cholesterol, and consumption of fat, particularly of saturated fat–the kind you find in meat and oils such as coconut and palm oils.

High fat consumption is also associated with cancer of the breast and colon. The main source of saturated fat in the human diet is the meat of ruminants, dairy products (high-fat dairy products such as whole milk), and hard margarine. Cholesterol is found only in foods of animal origin and particularly in eggs.

Fats

Fat is a source of essential fatty acids that help keep the body alive. Fats give the body structure, they are a carrier of fat-soluble vitamins such as A, D, E, and K, and they are necessary for metabolic functions.

The following is a list of oils beginning with what are considered the best oils, the healthiest oils to use.

Oils

Olive Oil – Olive oil contains 119 calories per tablespoon and is also highest in monounsaturated fat. One tablespoon contains 13.5 grams of fat, 9.9 of which come from unsaturated fat.

Canola Oil – Canola oil is also high in monounsaturated fat. One tablespoon contains 124 calories with a total of 14 grams of fat per tablespoon.

Safflower Oil – Safflower oil contains 120 calories per tablespoon and is high in polyunsaturated fat. This is also a good fat.

Other oils are not as high in unsaturated fat or polyunsaturated fats. Saturated fat is the least favorite type of fat. Limit your consumption of saturated fats.

Other oils that are often used in cooking are sesame, corn, soybean, peanut, vegetable, Crisco, palm and cottonseed, the latter of which are the least favorites.

How Much Oil Do We Need to Eat? Is There a Minimum?

We need one tablespoon of oil a day to avoid essential fatty acid deficiency. This is extremely uncommon and is rarely seen, even in the hospital setting, since most of the foods we eat contain some kind of fat. It is generally hard to avoid getting some. And as you can see, fat is essential.

Other foods high in fat are condiments such as mayonnaise and salad dressings, unless you choose fat-free or light varieties. To give you an idea of just how much fat these items contain, I have given a little breakdown.

Regular mayo   1 tablespoon 100 calories 11 grams fat

Low-fat mayo   1 tablespoon 25 calories 1 gram fat

Salad Dressing

Italian	1 T	60 calories	7.1 grams fat
Light Italian	1 T	16 calories	1.5 grams fat
Thousand Island	1 T	59 calories	5.6 grams fat
Light Thousand Island	1 T	24 calories	1.6 grams fat

Fat-free dressings are even lower in calories and are often completely fat-free.

Fat gives satiety.

What about butter? Which is better, butter or margarine? My thoughts are that butter is better. It is better-tasting and contains less trans fat. Butter tastes better and melts better, but do not use lots of it. It has been around forever, and cooks like using it.

One tablespoon of butter contains 100 calories, 11 grams fat, and 31 milligrams cholesterol.

One tablespoon of margarine contains 102 calories, 11.4 grams fat, and no cholesterol.

If cholesterol is an issue, I suggest watching the amount of fat you eat and limiting the high-cholesterol foods, but a little butter will not kill you.

TOO MUCH FAT is the problem, not the cholesterol. Along with all the fat, you get cholesterol. So if you end up eating more margarine because it has no cholesterol, you will end up eating more fat, thereby making up for the extra cholesterol intake by producing more on your own. Our bodies make cholesterol naturally. Whatever you do not eat, your body will make. Cholesterol is not an essential nutrient because our bodies make it, but it has some major functions within our bodies.

The following is a list of the 50 fattiest foods.

The 50 Fattiest Foods

Butter

Oils (olive, peanut, corn, soybean, safflower, sesame)

Olives

Pine nuts

Macadamia nuts

Chocolate

Salad dressings

Brazil nuts

Cream cheese

Coconut meat

Mayonnaise

Avocados

Lamb, rib chops, prime, broiled

Almonds

Beef, rib choice

Sausage

Luncheon meat

Shortening, all types

Margarine

Meat fat

Cream

Light whipping cream

Coconut milk

Pecans

Hazelnuts

Creamer

Sour cream

Walnuts

Pate de foie gras

Sunflower seeds

Sesame butter

Deviled ham

Beef, T-bone steak, choice

Beef, porterhouse steak, choice

Chapter 5: Carbohydrates

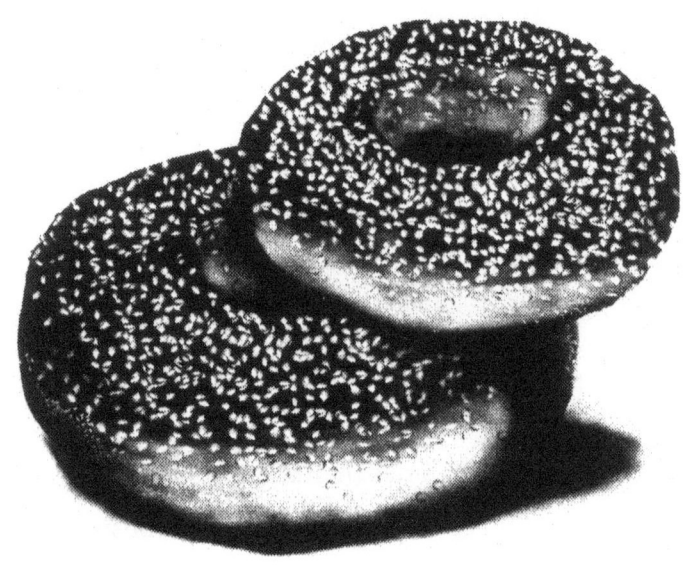

Carbohydrates-

One serving of a carbohydrate contains anywhere
between 70 calories and 160 calories. Some examples
might include half a bagel, half of a baked potato,
or even a slice of bread. A 202-gram baked potato
contains 220 calories, so half a potato is considered 1
serving.

Always remember that a carbohydrate's main goal is
to provide energy.

The following is a list of commonly eaten
carbohydrates that may even be considered staples for
some people.

Angel food cake (1 small piece) 137 calories
Bagel, plain 93.5 calories (half a small 3 oz. bagel)
Bagel, 3 oz. 120 calories (a large bagel is considered
2 servings)
Bread, 1 slice 70 calories – 110 calories

English muffin 120 calories

Pita 79 calories

Hot dog bun 129 calories

Pasta 1 serving (2 oz.) 210 calories

White rice 200 calories per cup, cooked

½ cup of rice is considered 1 serving

½ white potato baked w/skin 110 calories

½ sweet potato (1 small) 117 calories

Tortilla one 8" 115 calories

Pancakes

cereal

All Bran ½ cup 107 calories

Cheerios 1 cup 110 calories

Corn Flakes 1 cup 96 calories

Shredded Wheat ½ cup 76 calories

Grape Nuts ¼ cup 97 calories

Graham crackers (3) 88 calories

Popcorn 4 cups air-popped 122 calories (no added oil)

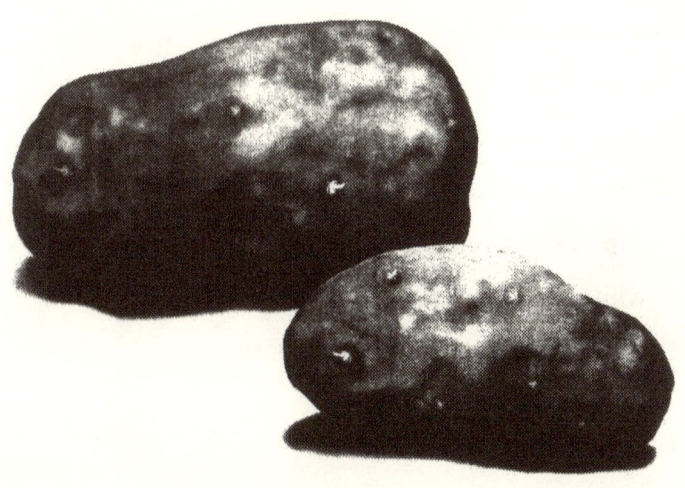

With carbohydrates, the best advice is to watch your portion sizes. With small portions, you are more likely to be hungry for your next meal and less likely to become overly full and uncomfortable. Similar to fat and sugar overeating, even nonfat to low-fat carbohydrates can turn to fat. It does not matter what the source is; if you have too much energy intake, your body converts the extra energy to storage, which is better known as fat for a rainy day.

The next examples are of familiar candy bars. I just wanted to show you how many calories they contain and what you can get nutrient-wise in place of your favorite junky snack.

Baby Ruth – 162 calories

Butterfinger – 211 calories

M&M's – 208 calories

Mars Bar – 242 calories

Snickers – 276 calories (a turkey sandwich is equal in calories!)

Skittles (mainly sugar) – 142 calories

Chapter 6: Fruit

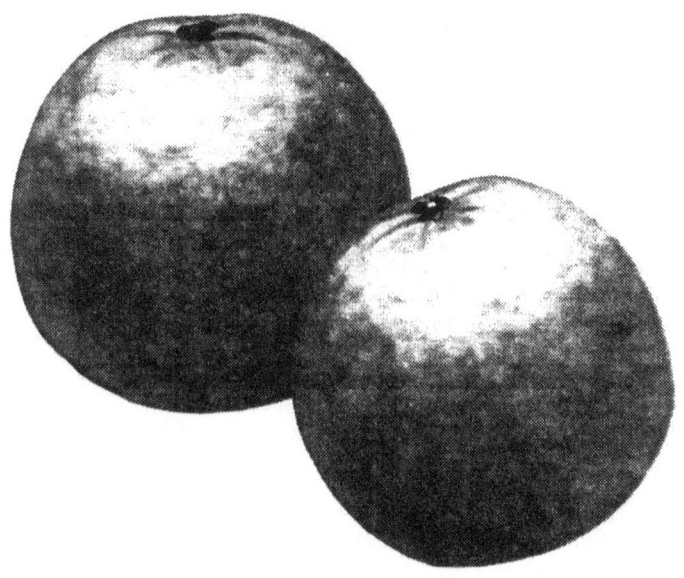

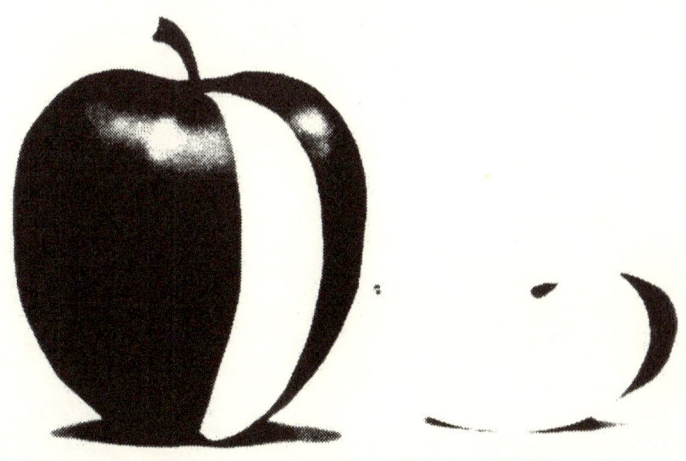

Fruit, like vegetables, provides essential vitamins and minerals. Some are high in vitamin C; others are high in vitamin A. Citrus fruits generally are a great source of vitamin C. Kiwi fruit is also high in vitamin C. Cantaloupe is high in vitamin A.

One serving of fruit might be considered ½ of a large apple.
One serving of a banana is ½ of a large banana.

Remember, serving sizes are important to consider. Even fruit, if eaten in large quantities, can contribute to fat storage. Try to eat at least five servings of fruit a day. For example, this might consist of an apple, a banana, and a small orange. It does not mean five pieces of fruit the way it sounds. It is five servings of fruit unless they are very small pieces of fruit.

The following is a list of fruits and their caloric content along with a suggested serving size.

Apple 1 small 81 calories or ½ a medium apple

Apple, dried 10 rings 155 calories

Applesauce ½ cup 97 calories

Apricots 3 small 51 calories

Apricots, dried 5 83 calories

Avocado 1 306 calories (30 grams of fat) (generally eaten by slices)

Banana 1 small 105 calories or ½ a large banana

Blackberries ½ cup 37 calories

Blueberries 1 cup 82 calories

Blueberries, frozen 1 cup 78 calories

Cherries (sweet) 10 49 calories

Crabapples 1 cup 83 calories

Cranberries 1 cup whole 46 calories

Cranberry sauce, sweetened ½ cup 209 calories

Currants ½ cup 36 calories

Dates 10 228 calories

Elderberries 1 cup 105 calories

Figs 1 medium 37 calories

Kiwifruit 1 76 calories

Kumquat 1 12 calories

Lemon w/peel 1 22 calories – w/o peel 17 calories

Lime 1 20 calories

Litchi fruit 1 6 calories

Loganberries, frozen 1 cup 80 calories

Mango 1 medium 135 calories

Melon, cantaloupe ½ 94 calories

Melon, casaba 1/1 (a slice) 43 calories

Melon, honeydew 1 slice /10 129 calories

Nectarine 1 67 calories

Orange 1 small 62 calories

Papaya 1 117 calories

Passion fruit 1 18 calories

Peach 1 small 37 calories

Peaches, canned ½ cup 60 calories

Pear 1 98 calories

Persimmon, Japanese 118 calories

Persimmon, native small 32 calories

Pineapple 1 slice 42 calories

Plantain 1 218 calories

Plum 1 small 36 calories

Pomegranate 1 104 calories

Prickly pear 1 42 calories

Prunes dried 10 201 calories

Raisins 1 cup 428 calories

Raspberries 1 cup 61 calories

Strawberries 1 cup 149 calories

Tangerine 1 small 37 calories

Watermelon 1/16 152 calories

Fruit juices such as orange juice can provide calcium
(which has been added) in addition to vitamins.
Juices, however, tend to be caloric substitutes for
the fruit you may wish to eat instead of drink. For
example, one 8–oz. glass of orange juice contains 112
calories whereas 1 small orange contains 62 calories
and is a good source of vitamin C and calcium on its
own along with folate and magnesium. It is always
better to eat your fruit than drink it. Drinking fruit
juices can raise your blood sugar a lot more quickly
than eating fruit. It often takes a little bit more time
and energy to eat your fruit, but it's the experience
and entertainment that makes it all the better.

Chapter 7: Vegetables

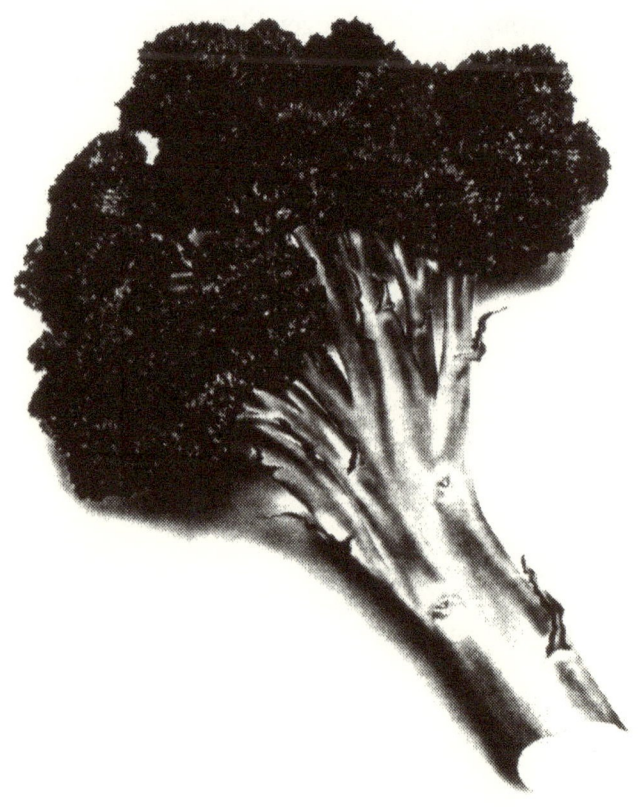

Vegetables-

Vegetables contain essential vitamins and minerals.
They average between 20 and 45 calories per serving.
A general rule to remember is that the orange
vegetables tend to contain higher amounts of vitamin
A and more antioxidants.

The following is a list of vegetables to include in
your diet. There are plenty to choose from. A normal
serving size ranges from ½ a cup to 1 cup.

Asparagus	Broccoli
Cauliflower	Peas
Green pepper	Red pepper
Yellow pepper	Mushrooms
Corn (often considered a carbohydrate because of the starch content)	Artichoke
Arugula	Beets
Brussels sprouts	Cabbage
Bok choy	Celery
Carrots	Swiss chard
Chives	Collard greens (high in vitamins A and K)
Cucumber	Dandelion
Eggplant	Endive
Fennel (high in vitamin A)	French beans
Garlic	Gingerroot
Green beans	Snap peas
Kale	Kohlrabi
Leeks	Romaine lettuce
Head (iceberg) lettuce (little nutrients at all)	Spinach
Okra	Onions
Parsley	Pimentos
Pumpkin	Radicchio
Radish	Ratatouille
Rhubarb	Seaweed
Shallots	Snow peas

Squash (winter, acorn, summer)	butternut
Turnip	Turnip greens
Water chestnuts	Watercress
Yellow beans	Yam (also considered like a carbohydrate because of starchy content)

Chapter 8: Alcohol

Alcohol-

Alcohol is a source of energy (7 kcals/g), but it provides no nutritional value. In calculating food exchanges/choices, alcohol is counted as energy from fat; 1 serving of alcohol = 2 fats. Beer and wine also contain some carbohydrates, which should be counted in the total daily carbohydrate intake. Distilled liquors do not contain carbohydrates unless they are mixed with a carbohydrate-containing beverage (e.g., cranberry juice or orange juice such as a cranberry absolute or a screwdriver).

Certain people should be careful with alcohol such as those with hypertriglycemia, pancreatitis, gastritis, neuropathy, and certain types of kidney and heart disease. Anyone experiencing hypoglycemia and women during pregnancy and while breast–feeding should avoid alcohol.

Alcohol can be caloric. It is not fat-free. If you are watching your weight, try drinking lower calorie drinks such as light beer, or a Tom Collins, a Bloody Mary, or a gin and tonic.

The following is a list of popular drinks and their caloric breakdown.

Alexander	179 kcals
Bacardi	118 kcals
Black Russian	255 kcals
Bloody Mary	123 kcals
Bourbon w/scotch or soda	105 kcals
Daiquiri	113 kcals
Gibson	158 kcals
Gin and tonic	171 kcals
Gimlet	132 kcals
Grasshopper	164 kcals
Mai Tai	310 kcals
Manhattan	127 kcals
Margarita	170 kcals
Martini	158 kcals
Mint Julep	156 kcals
Old Fashioned	155 kcals
Pina Colada	231 kcals
Rum and Coke	160 kcals
Screwdriver	182 kcals
Singapore Sling	228 kcals
Sloe Gin Fizz	121 kcals
Stinger	282 kcals
Tequila Sunrise	189 kcals
Tom Collins	121 kcals

White Russian	268 kcals
Wine Cooler	101 kcals
Wine 3 ½ oz.	70 kcals
Dessert Wine	153 kcals
Beer 12 oz.	151 kcals
Light Beer	101 kcals

Even alone, liquor can be caloric.

See the following examples.

1 jigger/42 grams

Gin	110 kcals
Rum	97 kcals
Vodka	97 kcals
Whiskey	105 kcals
Liqueur	74 kcals

Chapter 9: Diabetes

Diabetes-

Diabetes is also known as diabetes mellitus. Diabetes is characterized by a failure of the body to control energy production. Something has gone metabolically wrong. There are two types of diabetes: type 1 and type 2.

Type 1 diabetes is genetically inherited. This type usually runs in the family. Type 2 diabetes is typically seen in the elder population, but it is currently on the rise in children as well. Too much sugar and fat intake over a matter of time is unhealthful at any age.

In diabetes, the cells metabolize glucose (sugar) ineffectively with secondary effect on lipid and protein metabolism.

An analogy to what is happening metabolically when someone is diagnosed with diabetes is to think of an almost-empty street with several people wandering around, trying to get inside and off the street. They are trying to go into doors, either stores or homes, but the doors are locked, and they cannot get in. The people end up hanging around, possibly clogging up the street.

The people are the sugars, and the sugars want to go to your cells where your body will recognize them and utilize them as energy. Your body is unable to utilize this energy when it is roaming around in your blood vessels. A functioning system will accept the sugars, even in excess, and escort the sugars into your cells with insulin being the escort (or like the key to the doors). When the sugars do not get inside your cells, your body does not think it has energy available, and it may go to other sources for energy.

This could be happening for numerous reasons, but most likely, a diabetic person's body is not producing enough insulin required to help escort the passage of glucose to the cells. One reason for this inability to produce insulin may be thought of as a toy that gets used too many times and just shuts down and breaks.

Diabetes can lead to serious long-term disabilities, beginning with insulin shots (which are required to help control one's own blood sugar levels) to amputations (which occur due to the inefficiency of oxygenated blood to get to body parts, which occurs due to poor circulation). Other complications associated with diabetes include cardiovascular disease, renal disease, and ultimately renal failure.

Severe buildup of fat in large blood vessels (a.k.a. atherosclerosis) can occlude the vessels and reduce circulation to a body part. An occlusion, particularly in the legs and feet of diabetics, can lead to intermittent claudication, which may lead to the amputation of a limb, toe, or foot.

Hyperglycemia, which is defined as elevated blood sugar levels, is a result of an absolute or relative deficiency of insulin.

There are many people who control their diabetes by diet alone by watching their sugar and carbohydrate intake, and there are those that require insulin injections. What is known is that you can control your destiny, especially if diabetes does not run in your family. Type 2 diabetes is avoidable. By watching your fat and sugar/carbohydrate intake, you help maintain a healthy, functioning body over a lifetime.

Obesity is the most important risk factor in non-insulin diabetics. In countries where obesity is uncommon, diabetes is less common. Experts say obesity causes insulin resistance. And weight loss, even just 10 percent of body fat, can correct the problem. Weight loss is even more effective than insulin-lowering drugs. The author of a book titled *Syndrome X* points out that insulin resistance is a silent killer. And although insulin is released to process carbohydrates and can, at the same time, promote the storage of fat, it will do the latter only when more calories are consumed than are used by the body. In other words, it is neither insulin nor carbohydrates that make people fat: It is an excess of calories. When more calories are consumed than used, it is excess calories from fat that the body places in storage first. This is a very important point, and that is why it is essential that you know just how much you should eat a day.

People with diabetes and high blood pressure risk not only dying early, but they tend to start losing mental abilities in middle age, researchers say. A finding published in the journal *Neurology* said that it was important to start treating these two conditions, which are common in the United States and other developed countries, as early as possible. The study tested more than 10,000 people from across the United States who ranged in age from 47 to 70 years old. The researchers followed up six years later. The study showed that diabetes and hypertension were major risk factors for losing cognitive function over the six years.

Chapter 10: Cholesterol

Cholesterol-

What is it? Is it really something we need to worry about? What foods is it found in? And did you know that your body makes its own?

Cholesterol is not considered an essential nutrient. It is known as the silent killer, and it is associated with higher risks of heart disease. Elevated levels of cholesterol, smoking, and hypertension are indications of greater heart disease risk.

Cholesterol is an essential metabolite in animal cells but not in plant cells. This means that it is not found in plants whatsoever. When they advertise peanut butter without cholesterol, keep in mind that the peanuts never had it to begin with. Avocados are high in fat, but they contain no cholesterol. Cholesterol has several functions in the body.

Structurally, cholesterol modulates membrane fluidity and permeability of the cell to specific compounds. It is a component of the myelin sheath surrounding the axons of neurons (thereby playing an indirect role in the nervous system). Cholesterol is a precursor for the synthesis of bile acids and steroid hormones such as cortisone, estrogen, and testosterone.

Cholesterol is not essential in the diet because it can be synthesized from acetyl CoA by practically every tissue in the body. Its production in the body is regulated by what you eat. If you eat very little food containing cholesterol, your body will make the remainder of what it needs. One does not need to worry about being deficient in cholesterol. If you happen to eat foods with high amounts of cholesterol and fat, this may lead to excess fat production, thereby contributing to plaque buildup in your arteries.

Cholesterol is insoluble in water. A total of LDL, VLDL, and HDL l (good cholesterol) equals your total cholesterol count. Having a high HDL is considered good.

Cholesterol production can occur from overeating as well. Again, excess calories contribute to increased cholesterol counts.

Burning fewer calories reduces free radicals and extends life span. It is not yet known if caloric restriction would increase people's lifespan, but preliminary trials with monkeys look promising. Dr. Leonard Guarente, a biologist who studies aging at the Massachusetts Institute of Technology, recently showed how metabolism was directly linked to the cell's machinery for keeping its genes under control. Understanding the link between metabolism and aging would be significant, but there is certainly more to learn.

Bibliography

Brillat-Savarin, Jean Anthelme. The Physiology of
Taste or Meditations on Transcendental Gastronomy,
North Point Press, San Francisco, 1986.

Carper, Jean. Jean Carper's Total Nutrition Guide,
Bantam Books, New York, 1987.

Manual of Clinical Dietetics, 6th Edition, American
Dietetic Association, Chicago, IL, 2000.

Murray, Robert K., Mayes, Peter A., Granner, Daryl
K., Rodwell, Victor W. Harper's Biochemistry a
Lange Medical Book, 2nd Edition. Appleton and
Lange, Norwalk, Connecticut, 1990.

Williams, Sue Rodwell, Worhtington-Roberts, Bonnie S. Nutrition Throughout the Life Cycle, 2nd Edition. Mosby Year Book, St. Louis, MO, 1992.

Zeman, Frances, PhD, RD. Clinical Nutrition and Dietetics 2/e, Macmillan Publishing Company, New York, 1991.

About the Author

Jessica Cleary graduated from the University of California at Berkeley where she studied Nutrition and Food Science. Jessica has worked as a nutritionist in the fitness industry. She has also worked in the food industry and in clinical settings such as Northwestern Memorial Hospital and The Rehabilitation Institute of Chicago. Jessica currently resides in Chicago with her husband, Bill, and her son, Brendan.